Be The Best Medical Assistant:

A Customer Service Approach

T.L. Farley

ISBN-10:1983486787
ISBN-13:978-1983486784

DEDICATION

This book is dedicated to my husband Ryan who makes me laugh. Thank you for believing in me when I don't believe in myself. I love you.

.

CONTENTS

ACKNOWLEDGMENTS

I went through years of college courses earning my degree but it never appropriately prepared me for the work force. I was prepared with the understanding of terms and policies, I understood indications and contraindications, I had book knowledge of disease processes and diagnostics, but I had not received patient interaction training. Somewhere along the way, someone forgot to include training for the interactions I would have with real life patients. There is so much more to working in the health field as a service provider than just protocols and procedures. I want to give a general overview of the characteristics and skills you will need to succeed as an MA, beyond the clinical knowledge of procedures and policies. This book was designed to give you a collective understanding of the customer service aspect of working as a medical assistant (or any tech role) within the medical community.

Please know this is a basic overview and in no way, covers every circumstance or aspect of the customer service portion of health care. However, it does give a clear understanding of the qualities that will be important for you to consider when pursuing your career goals.

I wish you the best of luck in your future endeavors and hope this will help clarify for you the inherent qualities that an individual should possess or work to hone to succeed in this field. May your purpose be revealed to you in the pages of this book.

1 WHAT'S GOOD?

Ever wonder what makes someone good at their job while someone with the same qualifications and skill set can be so bad at theirs? Ever hear someone say, "He is good at his job but he has no personality"? Have you ever gone to a restaurant and had an inept server disappear and leave you at the mercy of seeking out another server for assistance? Have you ever gone to a store to make a purchase and the sales person treated you in a demeaning manor or ignored you altogether? When these instances occur do you ask yourself, *Is that allowed? I mean is this what the manager would want them to do? Is this ok? Is this how they treat their customers?* When these occasions happen in my own life I often question whether I know what the standards are for those services.

Perhaps the manager doesn't care if the waitress is nowhere to be found. Maybe the guy who is good at his job is the best there is and his personality doesn't matter to his employer. I have a saying I've been wanting to use but haven't had the opportunity present itself. The next time a service provider is rude to me I'm going to ask, "Do you volunteer?" I'm assuming they are not volunteering of course. Once they say they are not a volunteer, I plan to hit them with, "Oh, so you mean they pay you to be rude to their customers?" Pretty Good, huh?

A friend of mine had an experience recently at a well-known fast food chain. The food chain is implementing a new technology and insisted that my friend and his supervisor use their system. Instead of offering to take their orders at the cash register, as my friend and his supervisor had requested, the staff refused. When my friend asked to speak with a manager, the manager also insisted that they would no longer be taking orders at the register and advised them to use the new computerized system. It may seem like a small concern, to order from a computer as opposed to telling a cashier your order, but for older adults this new way is not as easy as we may think. Consider your grandparents or great-grandparents for this example. They do not navigate the new world of technology as easily as those of us who grew up using it. So while my friend could have easily used the computer system his supervisor could not. My friends' supervisor who was paying for the meal, announced their departure and his plan to have future meals at a competitor's restaurant. In addition, another patron who was standing behind them also announced her departure and agreed she would no longer purchase meals at this chain. She decided she would eat at the competitor's restaurant as well. At that all three potential customers left, resulting in a loss of sales for the food chain. Not to mention there are now three ex-patrons with negative reviews that will surely tell of their experience repeatedly. I used this example because this shows how one bad customer service experience can lead to financial loss for a company. In this example, the fast food chain had the ability to take orders from the register. However, when it was requested even the manager refused. In the end, the restaurant lost current sales and potential sales through a simple act of poor customer service.

It's frustrating to deal with people who lack the correct skills for the job they're in. Sometimes they have the skills but haven't been trained appropriately. Other times they just don't care about the job they are doing. In the field of customer service there is an old cliché, *"The customer is always right."* This idea isn't to be taken literally. It means that if it is within your ability to accommodate a customer request, for the sake of a positive customer service experience, it is always wise to err on the side of a satisfied customer. It does not mean break policies or laws. However, if you can take the order at the register, for the sake of customer satisfaction and potential return sales, take the order!

You're probably wondering why I am talking about customer service at a fast food restaurant. The answer is because customer service is important in any field where services are provided.

This includes the medical field. Many people forget that medical care is a service. How it is provided may depend on how the patient comes to you. For instance, a patient may come to the hospital several different ways. They may come by ambulance during an emergency. They may come voluntarily for a visit to the quick care for perhaps a sudden serious injury, a cut needing stitches. They may come with a friend or family member for an elective surgery, a procedure that's not necessary but may improve the quality of life and health. They may come for a general follow up for wound treatment. Perhaps they are having a follow up lab or other diagnostic testing. In every case mentioned the patient is coming to receive some type of service.

This is comparative to the fast food chain in that a customer may show up for a variety of meals. Perhaps breakfast, perhaps coffee, perhaps lunch, or dinner. Perhaps they are coming to eat with their team after a game, or a friend they haven't seen in ages, perhaps they are wanting a quick meal in a hurry. Whatever prompted the visit to the restaurant the patron is there for one basic reason, to receive a meal they will be paying for. The meal is a service the restaurant provides. Are you tracking with me?

The meal is provided as a service by the restaurant just as the hospital is providing health care services. I have always found it interesting how in the restaurant, retail, and sales industries we emphasize customer service, but the health care industry barely touches upon it.

The purpose of this book is to introduce important customer service standards to those beginning a career in the health care industry. In order to be the best you have to understand what the criteria is you will be judged by. You may think this stuff is common sense. In most cases these concepts should be inherent to the caregiver's nature. However, you may be surprised to find that is not always the case. In more recent years I have been increasingly discouraged with the type of customer service I have experienced in the retail, restaurant, sales, and health care industries. My hope is that a reminder of what excellent customer service looks like, specifically in the health care industry, will create a desire to increase the standards and achieve a level of excellence in customer service that has yet to be seen in health care.

2 WHO PAYS?

To become the best Medical Assistant you will first need to have a basic understanding of how the system works. Once you understand the basics you will have to commit yourself to taking consistent action and maintaining the level of expectation. The following chapter takes a look at your role and customer satisfaction play an important role in revenue.

Most of us don't think of our patients as customers. We think of them as patients. They need to see a physician who can help them manage their disease or recover from an illness. This is true. But it's also true that they pay for those services. You might argue that it is the insurance companies that are paying. I beg to differ, ask anyone who gets health insurance and taxes taken out of their weekly pay check and you will immediately understand we all pay for healthcare one way or another. The truth is that patients are paying for these services either out of pocket, through an insurance policy, through federal and or state assistance, or a privately funded organization. No matter how you look at it, someone must pay the bill for the services rendered. I hear the term "free care" get thrown around quite often. Let me clear this up for you, "free care" is not free. Someone must pay the bill. Free Care is medical service or treatment that is provided to the patient for free or at a low cost to the patient. However, there is still a cost that is incurred and will need to be paid by someone. The cost is deferred to another party in free care. This is either paid through government or state funded subsidies or private funded charities. Government and state funded programs are funded through the taxes that we pay either in state for example sales tax on registering our cars or federal taxes like when we file our tax returns. Privately funded programs are through individuals or organizations that have raised the money through donations and fundraisers to help pay a portion or all the costs. As with all sources, when the money runs out, so too the funding. Although the individuals offering free care may provide their services at no charge, the facility as well as supplies are not free. There is still a cost that is incurred when a patient is seen for a concern. Although the patient may not have the ability to pay for the service the equipment, supplies, and man hours that it took to treat the patient still needs to be paid.

The reason this is important to us as MA's is to understand that when a patient comes into our practice we are providing a service that they will be billed for and expected to pay (or will be paid by one of the aforementioned resources). The money that comes in from those patients allows the medical facilities the means to provide us with paychecks. This is an oversimplified explanation of the medical billing world. It's notable however because when we start to see our "patients" as customers we begin to understand that their satisfaction can ultimately affect our job security. As you begin to see each patient as a customer, even the most annoying patient will demand a level of respect that you perhaps didn't contemplate before. It's easy to get caught up in the idea that our patients need us, but , it is a symbiotic relationship. We need them just as much.

From this point on I will refer to our patients as

"customers". This will help us stay in the mind frame that we are in a position of service and not of power. I have seen MA's wait until the end of the day to call in a prescription for a customer. I've seen them speak rudely over the telephone to customers and I've seen them provide less than satisfactory service to customers. This is unacceptable in the service field. Like any salesman wanting to keep a routine customer and sales, it's important to provide the customer with what they are asking for. That doesn't mean breaking laws or procedures and policies. But the maxim "The customer is always right" should be understood. Of course, there are going to be times when your customer requests are not plausible and it's then you will need to practice diplomacy and patience. You will have to remember your customers are special. They are seeking a product that no money can buy, good health. Your job is to provide for them the product that allows them to get as close to good health as they can get and to make the journey to health an enjoyable one.

3 EXPERIENCE

I've asked customers over the years, "What is the worst part of coming to a doctor appointment?" Some say waiting, some say the bill, but hands down the most common answer has been the anticipation. Customers are nervous about what they will be told next. They are anxious about test results, or being told a condition has worsened. They want reassurance and peace of mind. Coming into a service center where the people make you feel like you are important and your health matters, can give them just that. It's especially comforting to know that if you must pay an expensive bill you got the best quality care possible.

Imagine that you are a customer. You show up to

have your office visit and the employees seem distracted, they are quick and uninterested in hearing your concerns. In the exam room the MA changes the old crinkly paper left there from the patient before you and asks you to have a seat. She quickly takes down the information she needs from you and leaves, telling you nothing. Eventually the doctor shows up and is just as quick to run through your information leaving you with unanswered questions. How will you feel when you receive the bill in the mail? How will you feel about having future appointments with the same office?

Now imagine that you are a customer. You show up to have your office visit and the employees are welcoming, they smile, they open doors, they sound happy to see you, they make you feel valued. They remember that you mentioned having a new puppy on your last visit 6 months ago. They ask you how things are going with the puppy while walking you to the exam room. Imagine that everyone has made you feel like this was an overall pleasant appointment. The MA is cordial while she gets the information she needs and lets you know the doctor is running on time, he will be in shortly. She smiles and asks that you bring a picture of your puppy in the next time you return, she is excited for you. Now imagine that you must keep coming back to be seen for this condition. Which place will you choose? Imagine that the second scenario charges $5.00 more for their visit, would you be discouraged to continue going?

Most people will pay the extra $5.00, because they are not just paying for the doctors expertise. They are paying for the whole experience and they want it to be as pleasant as it can be. The quality care and prompt service will likely make them feel like they have gotten their moneys worth.

This is where you come in. Your professionalism will add to the satisfaction of the customer. How quickly someone returns their calls, or sends in the necessary paperwork to their insurance company, all goes back to the people that work for the facility and helps to build a reputation. You are part of a sales team. If all the team's associates are on the same page the team will succeed.

4 ATTITUDE

In the next chapters we will explore some things you can do to create a positive experience for your customers. Creating a pleasant environment for your customers as you go through your day will eventually lead to the habit of providing good quality care. When you increase the quality of care you provide you will also increase the standard for others. Your team will notice your efforts and begin to increase their standards as well. Over time you will gain a reputation for providing the best care around and you may find yourself the MVP of your medical office.

One of the most important skills you can take with you in any field is a positive attitude. I call it a skill because if you aren't typically a positive person you can learn to be one. Practice. Learn all you can on having a positive outlook and practice it. No one wants to work with a negative Nellie. Your coworkers and your customers will thank you. If you are that one coworker who complains about everything and everyone, eventually it will catch up with you and you will most likely be overlooked for opportunities you may be most qualified for. A positive attitude goes a long way, especially in a health care setting. Your customers are often dealing with life threatening conditions, health concerns, and sometimes diseases. A good attitude, a smile and a kind word can brighten their day and ultimately lead to return visits due to the quality of the experience they had with you. Often customers will ask for MA's by name when they have had a good experience and managers will notice that customers are noticing you. An MA who complains about trivial life concerns and blames others for inconsistencies within the practice will appear shallow and unprofessional. Keep your bad day to yourself and if you have a legitimate gripe about something in the practice take it up with your practice manager. I have seen MA's talk about co-workers to customers. This does not create a professional environment. It may also make the customer feel uncomfortable as they have come for an appointment in which they want to feel confident that the office staff are professionals.

When working with coworkers a positive attitude can help make a bad day better. Remember it's easier to work with people you like. If you have ever worked with someone who complained constantly and always had a crisis to resolve, then you know how energy draining they can be. It's best to avoid a person like that as much as possible and try to keep your own positive perspective.

5 WAITING ROOM

When going to a doctor appointment most of us just show up and don't put much thought into what the staff had to do to prepare for our visit. Depending on where you work your responsibilities may require specific preparations prior to your customers arrival.

Depending on your role and office policies you may be required to gather records from your customers last office visits, procedures, emergency room visits, lab work and other pertinent health information. Sometimes you will need to call other practices in other states for information or lab work and records. All of this is important to know prior to your customer coming for their appointment. Gathering the information in a timely manner helps your office to be efficient, allows the doctors you work with to make appropriate treatment decisions, and allows your customer the comfort of knowing your office is providing quality care.

Once all the appropriate information is gathered familiarize yourself with the records. For instance, it is wise to read the current reason for their visit and their last office visit note prior to your customers arrival. This will help you to understand what they were last in for and whether it is an ongoing concern. It will also familiarize you with the customer prior to getting them from the waiting area. This may also provide an opportunity to ask a few follow-up questions to see how they have been doing since their last appointment. For example, they may have had a sinus infection the last time they were in, you may mention you remember they had a sinus infection at their last visit and ask how they have been feeling since. Remembering your customers in this way will help build a positive bond between you. They will feel that your care is sincere, and you are paying attention to their concerns. Also, the records you have may show that the customer hasn't had a doctor appointment in a few years. This is your opportunity to find out if they have been seen anywhere other than the places you have already requested information from. Sometimes out of state practices will not automatically send records and you may need to send a formal request for the information. It's best to find this out before the doctor goes in to see the patient, that way you can be working on getting the records as soon as possible. This will help you gather information to pass along to the doctor before he sees the customer.

A clean exam room is another priority before taking a customer from the waiting area. Make sure you have taken the time to straighten up the room. Wipe down the exam table, per company policies. Replace the exam table paper with fresh, wrinkle free paper. Look around, make sure there's a clean environment and if it isn't take the time to clean it. A fresh clean exam room reflects on you, not the cleaning staff. I have heard MA's say they are not cleaning an exam room because "it's not my job". That may be true, but it directly reflects on you and your office. Take a few minutes and make sure it is clean and presentable. Then go to your practice manager about your concerns with the overnight cleaning crew. You might be surprised to find out that some of the cleaning responsibilities are your job.

The final step before getting your customer from the waiting area is to make sure you have everything you need. Grab your stethoscope if you need it. Make sure you have the EKG cart in the room. If there are supplies the doctor needs you to stock, correct forms or equipment, make sure it is all there. There's nothing more frustrating than running around trying to find equipment while the customer and the doctor are waiting for you to do your job.

Finally, get your customer. Know who they are. Know how you are to ask for them. There are HIPPA regulations out there that require you to ask for your customers a certain way. Proceed in a manner that doesn't reveal unnecessary information to other customers in the waiting area. For instance, if you go to the waiting area and you call out "Susan?" and two women stand up, how will you determine which is the correct customer? Make sure you know what your policies are and be professional.

Once you have identified your customer introduce yourself. "Hi, I am _______, I am a ___________(medical assistant, cardiac tech, echo tech), welcome to our practice." You don't have to use this line exactly but use a friendly greeting that introduces who you are and what your title is. This will sometimes lead to further discussion about what you do and what your qualifications/experience is. Don't be offended or embarrassed. If you're new, tell them. They will be less likely to criticize you if they know you are still learning.

Once you have introduced yourself and have made your way through the pleasantries of the first impression, do your best. If the customer asks you questions you are unsure of you can say something like, "That is a question best answered by the doctor, I will let him know you asked." Remember to tell the doctor that they were asking so he will be prepared with an answer.

As you room your patient and proceed with the necessary assessments and collection of data continue to be polite while also being aware of time management. If a patient is telling you too much information or overly chatty be prepared to cut them off in the politest manner you can. You may say something like, "I'm sorry, I'm going to ask that you wait until the doctor is here, that way you won't have to tell your information more than once. He will want to hear it directly from you." Smile. Be kind and patient. There are some customers who will not take such subtle hints and you will need to be more direct. Let them know you do not want to keep the doctor waiting and you wish you had more time to talk with them. Most customers will understand and of course they do not want to keep the doctor waiting either.

When you leave the room, don't forget to let them know that the doctor is expected to be running on time or if there will be a short wait. They will appreciate knowing if the wait will be long or not. Either way it's good practice to let them know. Also, don't forget an exit statement, tell them it was a pleasure meeting them, or if they are a returning customer, it was nice to see them again. This will help support the feeling that you are hospitable, and their visit has been a pleasant one.

6 PERSONALITY

As you may already be aware, you are not going to like every person you meet. In return every person you meet is not going to like you. Sometimes you must smile and be polite even when they are not.

There are some customers who already have their minds made up about their experience. Don't take it personally. It helps to remember some of these folks have had several doctor appointments for symptoms they haven't been able to find causes for. Sometimes they have been around and around on the diagnostic merry go round with no diagnosis in sight. Remember they don't feel good and they are frustrated. Your compassion may change their attitude and may be the only good thing they've experienced so far. After all, it is not you they are angry at.

With that said, there are those customers who for whatever reason find it enjoyable to be disagreeable. You can't change that, but you can be professional. Provide the best quality care you are able and know that the customers attitude will be quick to reveal itself to others. In other words, if they are complaining about you to others, it wont be long until they are complaining about other aspects of their care as well. You will have to maintain your positive perspective. Be glad you practiced it. I have found that in time, most of these customers usually come to respect you and while they maintain their disagreeable attitude with others, your positive and professional demeaner can win some of them over.

People come in all personality types. There's the grumpy type that will always find something to complain about. When the appointment is perfect, they will complain about the taxi ride to the appointment. There's the appreciative type who is thankful for your help and all that you do. When you see their names on your schedule you will look forward to the visit. There's the condescending type who of course is more educated and more experienced than you. This personality will treat you as if you know nothing and are of no importance to their care. There is the fearful type. They will be afraid of the worst-case scenario and feel if it's going to happen to anyone, it'll happen to them. There's the irrational type, no matter what you do or how you do it, you will not please them as they are unwilling to be pleased. There's the unsure type who will ask you questions only the doctor is qualified to answer. This personality will call back several times after the doctor appointment to clarify exactly what the instructions were. Hopefully you get my point. As you become more familiar with customer personalities you will need to learn to "read" the customer and the appropriate way to relate to them. Some people use humor to cover up their fear, some people are angry that they are struggling with a health condition. You will need to learn to decipher what each customer needs from you in the time that you spend with them. Cracking jokes to a fearful customer will likely end in a poor response. This customer is not in the mood for jokes. A somber attitude when dealing with someone who is peppy and joking may result in the customer perceiving the appointment in a negative light as opposed to a joyful experience. Learn to read your customers.

As you gain confidence and experience in your field your customers will begin to look to you for specific guidance and comradery. Be sure you always follow protocol and policies. Customers will truly begin to value your care and sincerity. I have had customers come to visit me at my vacation spot, I've had customers bring me gifts of honey and other items. I even had a customer make me an entire lamp out of popsicle sticks! (Craft sticks, not actual popsicles he had eaten.) Treat others how you would want to be treated and they will recognize your efforts.

7 ACT

Honestly, there are going to be days you are not going to want to go to work. Everyone has those days. You may wake up with a cold or feel grouchy from a night of poor sleep, but you will still be expected to go to work and be the best you can be. This can be tough. As we all know, life happens. People divorce, children get in trouble, parents struggle, health can fail, whatever may be going on in your personal life you will have days where you are not going to be feeling it. You need to suck it up and act. True story. You may just have to fake it until you make it. Daily cheeriness is a commitment and doesn't come naturally to most of us. If you're one of those people that it does come easy to than you have certainly chosen the right field. For the rest of us, cheeriness needs to be practiced, and sometimes, faked. I'm not saying you have to be phony because your customers will see straight through that. I'm saying try to maintain a pleasant demeanor. It's ok to admit you're having a tough day as long as you stay polite and do your job.

Working with the public can be frustrating. People will push your buttons and say things that may be inappropriate or just rub you the wrong way in the moment. You must pretend it doesn't bother you and move on. Know that it will pass, and you will live to see a better day. This is where the positivity practice will come in handy. Be thankful for the job you have and the ability to work and receive a paycheck. Focus on the things that are worth focusing on. Remember the frustrating days happen no matter where you work or what field you work in. Even when you are doing exactly what you love you will struggle some days. This is completely normal and expected. If you're having a particularly difficult day, ask a co-worker if they might assist you so that you can take a quick break or lighten the load in exchange for your help with their work another day. If you maintain a strong work ethic the majority of the time, no one is going to complain when you have an off day.

8 WORK ETHIC

Work Ethic has become an ideology. Many companies are looking for reliable hard-working people to help their companies succeed but many employees seem to think the hard work stopped when they received the diploma. There used to be a time when hard-work was all you needed. However, in the push for the world to be more educated, degrees took the place of hard-work. Companies, and managers are now recognizing a degree doesn't necessarily mean you can handle the tasks at hand. In fact there are some people who are amazing at their jobs and have no degree to show for it. Instead they have years of experience. On the flip side, a degree might get you the job but it's your work ethic that will help you keep it. If you choose to apply this very simple guide, you will do well in your career. Currently there are few people who understand the importance of work ethic. It's important. It can make or break a career.

Be reliable. Only call out when necessary. Other employees will appreciate knowing you are going to be there when you are scheduled to be. This will create positive morale with coworkers. They will trust they can count on you. Coworkers that must cover your shift regularly will eventually feel resentful and angry that they are doing your work and theirs. Managers will get fed up with having to juggle employees to cover unexpected absences and tardiness. Managers will consider an employee they can rely on an asset. The ones they cannot rely on they will eventually let go.

Be flexible. If your coworker calls out for the 5th time in three weeks, know they won't be employed much longer. Understand that your manager is in a bind trying to fill the void with the people they have. Managers cannot fire employees at whim, there are policies and regulations in place that need to be followed before letting an employee go and hiring a new one. It takes time and you will be relied upon. In the meantime, take this opportunity to shine!

Be on time. Again, being late may require coworkers to cover part of your shift adding more work to theirs. This will again cause hard feelings and a make for a challenging work environment. When coworkers and managers know they can depend on you to do your job in its entirety they will respect you and appreciate you. Your promptness will promote feelings of reliability around your employment. Reliable employees add to a positive work environment. If you simply cannot get to work at the hours you are scheduled you should rethink your employment location or route of transportation. Maybe it's time to take a job that is closer or has more flexible hours.

Be honest. Communication is important. You will have to constantly be communicating with customers and other staff about what you are doing, when you did it, and whether it was done on time. Most computer systems keep records of time of messages and notices, fax machines, and other office equipment almost always post times that reports were printed, faxes were sent, messages were taken, etc., so be honest. If you forgot to do something admit it. Don't try to blame someone else for your mistakes. If you are working hard and going over and above, then one mistake will be overlooked. However, if you tend to make those mistakes often and blame or exaggerate about the circumstances regularly, you will lose trust with your employer. If you tend to exaggerate or tell half-truths, don't. Co-workers, customers, managers, and doctors will respect you for being honest and communicating with truthfulness. Employees who lie or try to blame others are easily figured out. No one wants to work with someone they can't trust.

This leads me to another form of communication, gossip. Refrain from being sucked into gossip. If you are someone who initiates it, learn to keep it to yourself. Gossiping can cause you to lose opportunities for supervisory positions as well as hurt your relationship with others. HIPPA regulations are very strict around what you can talk about and share with other customers and co-workers. Be aware of policies and when in doubt, don't say it out.

Be extra. My daughter likes to say, "You're so extra," when she feels I'm being dramatic about something. I'm not telling you to be dramatic, I'm telling you to do more than what is expected from you. Do your job over and above what is expected. For example, I would often send condolence cards to the families of customers who had passed away from the staff and doctor at our practice. It's those extra little things that let people know you care. Like I already mentioned, don't be that worker that says, "It's not my job." If it's truly beyond the scope of your certification or medical training than don't do it. But if your manager or a doctor is asking you to do something that you are able and qualified to do, just do it. You work for them remember? This will only work to your advantage. If additional training is involved, you will increase your skill set which increases your value as an employee. Having an employee that can do several jobs as opposed to several employees doing one job is a no brainer. Companies want people who are cross trained and reliable. Later, if there are layoffs and management have to decide to keep you or a coworker (that didn't do extra), you will be the one they keep.

Be willing to laugh. Have a sense of humor. Be willing to laugh at yourself and enjoy your co-workers and customers. Working with people in any capacity is an opportunity for humor. People are people no matter where you go. They are going to do things that are funny and say things that are funnier. Learn to enjoy it. I worked in a cardiology practice and had an elderly patient ask if he was supposed to take his pants off. He genuinely wasn't sure. I told him we only work above the waist. We shared a good laugh. Having a sense of humor with your co-workers can help you get through a tough day. Another time I noted that a customer had gained a considerable amount of weight since his last visit and asked if he had any changes to medications or lifestyle. He remarked that he was eating honey buns regularly. Later in the exam room he noted that marijuana had been legalized and told me that his neighbor smoked. He went on to describe how the smell would permeate his apartment. We joked that perhaps this was the reason he was eating honey buns more regularly. Having a sense of humor helps bring joy into your day. Your customers will notice.

9 FOLLOW THROUGH

I personally think "follow through" is an important quality in any field. Follow through is the continuation of an act to its completion. When a batter follows through with the baseball bat, he swings a complete swing, so the bat hits the ball and then continues to follow through the rest of the swing.

When a customer asks you to call in a refill for a prescription and you say you will do it, do it. The job isn't complete because you told them you would do it, it's complete once it is done and you have called the patient back to let them know it has been done. That is follow through. It's easy to get busy and forget to do something so simple. But it reflects on you when it is not done and makes you appear to your customers as if you are inept. Keep a note pad with you and write down things you need to do. As you do them cross them off the list. It will help you remember the things you need to get done and your customers and managers will appreciate your efficiency.

Think of it this way, a friend makes plans to be at your house by a certain time. You take a shower and get dressed and are anticipating their arrival. You wait and wait and wait some more. Eventually you call your friend and get their voice message. You leave a message and wait a few hours longer. After a bit you become worried. Perhaps something has happened to your friend so you call them again. This time your friend answers and says they will have to call you back. Again you wait. When your not so very good friend finally calls you back she tells you she's not going to be able to make it after all. Now you have spent your day waiting and worrying when you could have had a more productive and enjoyable day.

When you tell a customer that you will look into something for them, do it. If it's a question for the doctor, call the patient and let them know he hasn't gotten to it yet and you will call them as soon as he does. If you can't get to it that day call them and let them know you will do it the following day, so they know that you are working on getting them an answer. Customers will appreciate that you took the time to keep them in the loop. They do not want to sit around waiting for a phone call they are never going to get.

In the MA world, you may find a lot of your time is spent trying to get back to customers with answers regarding insurance coverage on their prescriptions, or lab results. This is important information for the customers. Their medication can be a matter of life or death in some cases. Try to remember the importance of your part in making sure they have what they need on their journey to health.

10 ASK

This is another important aspect of being the best you can be. Ask questions. Learn. If you don't understand something, be honest, ask someone to explain it to you. Ask for further training if you can't do something correctly. Ask the doctors what you can do better. If you work with one specifically, ask how they prefer things done. The more you ask the more you know. It's better than finding out at review time that you are not cutting it.

Ask to observe others. Observe co-workers, what do they do well, what can you do better? Integrate what they do well with what you do well. If there are procedures or practices within your field that you are unfamiliar with, ask if you can watch one. Often managers will allow this to help you gain a better understanding of the services your office provides. Doctors will appreciate you taking the time to see them in action and understand what it is they do. The more you know about the procedures the better you will be able to answer patient questions and understand processes within the practice.

Ask for training. Get any training you can, whether it's for your immediate use or to cover another department in a pinch. The more training you have, the more skills you have, the more marketable you are. The more marketable you are, the more valuable you are as an employee. The more valuable you are the more likely you are to maintain employment and the more options you will have for employment in other areas. All of this could potentially lead to more money in your paycheck and opportunities for supervisory positions.

Ask for reimbursement and wage increases. When you have completed a new certification and a new training you are now more qualified. It doesn't hurt to ask your manager for potential pay increase to reflect your more marketable skills. Don't be afraid to ask. The worst they will do is say no. Of course, be professional as well. Don't gripe and complain to others if you do not get the pay increase. Remember they can't reimburse for every little thing, but a major certification should certainly qualify you for a potential raise, if not today, during your annual review.

It's important to ask questions. Don't be afraid to look dumb, the only way you will understand is if you ask. Get the answers you need so you can be better than you were before.

FINAL THOUGHT

Most importantly take care of yourself. Know when to say no. Set boundaries. Know your scope of practice so you are not practicing outside of them. Be confident enough to say you're not comfortable with something. Get plenty of rest, eat right, and get exercise. You cannot take care of others if you are too sick to take care of yourself. Enjoy your journey. Caring for others is a career that not everyone is cut out for. You will feel exhausted one day and exuberant on another. Take comfort in knowing that what you do matters, even when it doesn't feel like it does. You really are making a difference in the life of those you meet. The quality of care you give reflects on you as well as on the company you are working for. More importantly, the quality of care you give impacts and at times influences those you are giving it to.

Trust me when I tell you, if you work to consistently implement the concepts discussed here, your life will be richly impacted as well. You will get to meet interesting people doing interesting things. I've met owners of breweries, actresses, singers, war heroes, concentration camp survivors, political figures, basketball players, and many others. They have shared their stories with me and encouraged me to be my best. Some I have called friends and others blessings. Some still stay in contact with me. Some of them have been my biggest supporters in the journey that I have taken and some of them have been even bigger inspirations to the journey I am still on.

I wish you the greatest success and hope all who read this book will take the opportunity to show gratitude to those who have helped you become who you are at this moment. May this book be one you are thankful for as it helps you become who you want to be in the future.

About the Author

Tawny is a veteran in customer service. She worked in cardiology for 10 years, the medical field for 20, and customer service since she was a teenager. Her first job was working at a swim suit store where she learned her first lessons in customer service. She believes the little things count when it comes to good customer service. She addresses this subject because she believes providing excellence in customer service is a dying ideology.

www.ingramcontent.com/pod-product-compliance
Lightning Source LLC
Chambersburg PA
CBHW071242220526
45468CB00002B/969

9781983486784